YOGIC COOKING

of related interest

Mudras of India
A Comprehensive Guide to the Hand
Gestures of Yoga and Indian Dance
Cain Carroll and Revital Carroll
Foreword by Dr. David Frawley
ISBN 978 1 84819 084 9 (hardback)
ISBN 978 1 84819 109 9 (paperback)
eISBN 978 0 85701 067 4

Mudras of Yoga
72 Hand Gestures for Healing and Spiritual Growth
Cain Carroll
With Revital Carroll
Card Set
ISBN 978 1 84819 176 1
eISBN 978 0 85701 143 5

Mudras of Indian Dance
52 Hand Gestures for Artistic Expression
Revital Carroll
With Cain Carroll
Card Set
ISBN 978 1 84819 175 4
eISBN 978 0 85701 142 8

Eat to Get Younger
Tackling inflammation and other ageing
processes for a longer, healthier life
Lorraine Nicolle and Christine Bailey
ISBN 978 1 84819 179 2
eISBN 978 0 85701 125 1

Make Yourself Better
A Practical Guide to Restoring Your Body's
Wellbeing through Ancient Medicine
Philip Weeks
ISBN 978 1 84819 012 2
eISBN 978 0 85701 077 3

YOGIC COOKING

Nutritious Vegetarian Food

Compiled by Garuda Hellas

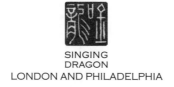

SINGING
DRAGON
LONDON AND PHILADELPHIA

This edition published in 2015
by Singing Dragon
an imprint of Jessica Kingsley Publishers
73 Collier Street
London N1 9BE, UK
and
400 Market Street, Suite 400
Philadelphia, PA 19106, USA

www.singingdragon.com

First published in 2013 by Garuda Hellas, Thessaloniki, Greece

Copyright © Garuda Hellas 2013, 2015

Front cover image source: Veer

Library of Congress Cataloging in Publication Data
A CIP catalog record for this book is available from the Library of Congress

British Library Cataloguing in Publication Data
A CIP catalogue record for this book is available from the British Library

ISBN 978 1 84819 249 2
eISBN 978 0 85701 195 4

Printed and bound in Great Britain

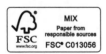

MIX
Paper from
responsible sources
FSC
www.fsc.org
FSC® C013056

Dedicated to Swami Satyananda, Swami Niranjanananda and Swami Sivamurti for their continuous inspiration.

A heartfelt thank you to Satyanandashram Hellas (www.satyanandayoga.gr), to Swami Aparokshananda and to Swami Jnanamudrananda for their generous service in the ashram kitchen over many years and for their valuable contribution and thoughtful guidance in the creation of this long-awaited cookbook.

This book is a practical demonstration of how one can do wonders with simple ingredients, not only in terms of taste, but also in regards to one's health, quality of thoughts and energy.

The recipes in this book come from the Bihar School of Yoga, Munger, India (www.yogavision.net), which is our source, and from Satyanandashram Hellas, Greece, which has adapted some Greek-style vegetarian dishes for the yogic lifestyle.

CONTENTS

YOGIC COOKING

The yogic diet is primarily a vegetarian one that also includes some dairy products, in particular milk, yogurt and cheese. It consists of plant-based foods that are wholesome and fresh, without preservatives and chemical additives.

What are the benefits of such a diet? What do we gain when we include, for example, the combination of "Sabji, rice and dhal" in our daily eating habits?

Dhal is legumes (usually split peas, red lentils or mung beans) cooked in combination with certain condiments, which help to accelerate the digestive process.

Sabji is vegetables, also cooked with the same combination of condiments. Seasonal vegetables are used as they are fresh, more readily available and better value for money.

Meat-eaters object to an exclusively plant-based diet, claiming that we cannot derive the proteins we need from just eating fruit and vegetables.

Our body needs amino acids to synthesize the protein. Most of the total amino acids the human body needs, 22 altogether, can be synthesized through the breaking down of food. There are, however, eight amino acids that the body is not able to synthesize and these have to be digested from certain foods that already contain them intact. People who eat meat, fish, eggs and animal products (milk, yogurt, etc.) are not deficient in these eight particular amino acids. People who follow a yogic diet, on the other hand, need to consume a combination of legumes, cereals and vegetables, prepared with certain condiments, on a daily basis in order to take in this chain of eight essential amino acids.

Since ancient times yoga practitioners have found that a diet consisting of fresh and cooked vegetables, combined with cereals and legumes and prepared using special condiments, is the ideal. Spices are not merely for seasoning and adding flavour – they contain elements that are identical to the enzymes of the body and therefore help digestion. Some examples of these are: coriander, anise, cumin, mustard seeds, turmeric, black pepper and cardamom.

An excellent example of a meal at the ashram is the combination of rice (grain) and dhal (pulse soup). By eating rice and dhal daily, we receive all of the eight essential amino acids.

Our body also needs vitamins and minerals. These we derive mainly from vegetables (cooked as sabji). It is important to consume a variety of vegetables so our body gets everything it wants and needs to maintain itself. When we decide to follow a vegetarian diet, we need to ensure that we get the necessary vitamin B12 and iron that our body requires.

Another significant benefit of a yogic diet is that the food is digested easily. This is important because it means that we do not spend all our energy digesting; instead we are free to use our energy to create, to produce, and to live life to the full.

"It is better to cook your food in the pot rather than in the stomach. The combination of temperature with the spices makes the food more digestible, so less energy is consumed during digestion."

SWAMI SATYANANDA

YOGA AND VEGETARIANISM

The general impression is that vegetarianism is an integral part of yoga. However, yoga does not impose dietary restrictions on anybody; it simply proposes a nutritious, toxin-free diet. Yoga aims to cultivate physical, mental and emotional balance in individuals, so that they can experience the higher states of their being. This can be achieved with a balanced vegetarian diet that includes all the essential minerals and vitamins.

Diet is adjusted according to the season, our state of health and our activities. What and how much we eat depends on whether we sit for long hours in meditation or do dynamic asanas or a lot of karma yoga, or whether we are in full health or have a common cold, and so on and so forth.

In every part of the world, everyone adapts their diet according to the prevailing climatic and geographical conditions. That is why the diet of those living in cold climates, such as Scandinavia and Alaska, contains more animal foods, while nearer the equator, where the climate is much warmer, lighter diets that are rich in vegetables and fruits are consumed.

Archimedes and Pythagoras, along with other ancient Greeks, believed that vegetarianism brought peace and harmony to both the body and the mind, whereas meat-eating fuelled inner tension, producing disharmony and fervent obsession.

"Through much trial and error yogis came to the conclusion that some foods are unsuitable for the human body. If you analyze the secretions of the digestive tract, the gums, the teeth and the secretions of the salivary glands, if you examine the strength of the mucous membranes along the length of the small and large intestine and make a comparison with other carnivores and animals that feed on raw nuts and seeds, you will see that there is a difference. The length of our intestines is evidence that the human body should consume cooked, vegetarian food. A natural, macrobiotic diet is ideal."

SWAMI SATYANANDA

"It is not necessary to abandon meat-eating in order to do yoga. If you practise regularly, you will see that after a while meat will abandon you. I recommend a diet for your better health and to speed up your evolution. You will see and feel the change at a physical level and you will also observe a mental alertness, a brightness and sensitivity. But it is not enough to stop eating meat. If you eat nutritious food and you use the increased energy for slander, cheating or lies, then it is wasted. It is better if a person has unhealthy eating habits but uses their energy for a good cause. Take care of your diet, control your speech, observe your thoughts."

SWAMI SAYANANDA

TYPES OF VEGETARIANS

We come across vegetarians with different habits:

- Vegans: do not consume any animals or animal-derived products (milk, cheese, yogurt, eggs).

- Lacto vegetarians: as well as fruits and vegetables, they also consume dairy products but not eggs, or cheeses which contain animal rennet.

- Vegetarians: also consume dairy products and eggs.

When someone decides to become a vegetarian, they are likely to be confronted with different views and maybe even objections from friends and relatives. At first, they may not know how to substitute animal with vegetable protein. But then, any fresh start in life is a period of discovering and creating new habits.

This cookbook is a perfect companion to help you to get acquainted with yogic recipes and to learn to cook them as they are prepared in an ashram, where people live a traditional yogic lifestyle.

Hari Om
The best way to learn yogic
cooking is to come and
Spend some time
in the
ashram.

We look forward to having
you
with
us.

Sivani C.

THE PSYCHOLOGY OF COOKING

A good diet is important for the health of the body, as well as of the mind. Food influences the state of our mind not only through its chemical effect, but also through its vibrations. The state of the mind at the time of preparation and consumption also affects both the vibrations of the food and the biochemical composition of our digestive system.

When we have energy we feel better and our thoughts are positive. On the other hand, when our energy is low, we feel down and we see the things around us in a negative light. That is why in yoga there is an emphasis on the vital energy, or prana, that we receive from the food we eat and the environment around us.

We can further activate our food by preparing it with our hands. It also helps to have positive thoughts, sing or listen to mantras (beneficial sound vibrations), enjoy and take pleasure in the process, think kind and caring thoughts of the people who will receive the food, so that the meal becomes an offering and an act of love.

Another important factor in the preparation of our food is cleanliness. The kitchen needs to be clean and tidy before, during and after the cooking of each meal. In this way, we show our respect to both the space in which we do our cooking and the utensils we use.

We need to be relaxed during meals, otherwise the enzymes necessary for digestion are not released, which means that many of the nutrients are not absorbed. These days, the necessity to regularly refuel our stomachs may feel like a chore, and every now and then we may complain about this bodily need. Nevertheless, at mealtimes we should make a conscious effort to be relaxed, focus on the present and, above all, feel grateful for the food we have in front of us.

Finally, yoga proposes the ideal position for digesting our food when we finish our meal. Vajrasana (thunderbolt or zen pose) is particularly beneficial for improving the function of the digestive system in a natural way.

Vajrasana

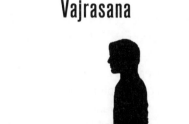

Kneel on the floor. Bring the big toes together and separate the heels. Lower the buttocks onto the inside surface of the feet with the heels touching the sides of the hips. Place the hands on the knees, palms down. The back and head should be straight but not tense. Avoid excessive backward arching of the spine. Close your eyes, relax the arms and the whole body. Breathe normally and fix the attention on the flow of air passing in and out of the nostrils. (Taken from *Asana Pranayama Mudra Bandha* by Swami Satyananda Saraswati, Yoga Publications Trust, Munger, Bihar, India.)

VITAMINS AND MINERALS

Vitamins and minerals are our essential allies. For instance, on a daily basis we need vitamins A, B, C, D, E and the following minerals: calcium, phosphorus, magnesium, potassium, sodium and iron. The question that hovers over every aspiring vegetarian is: "If I become a vegetarian, where will I get the nutrients found in meat, fish, etc.?" But we now know that the different vegetables contain high concentrations of many of the vitamins and minerals that our body needs.

The following tables summarize which plant-foods contain those vitamins and minerals, and explain what they are good for.

Vitamins

Vitamins	What they are good for	Where they are found
A	Essential in the formation and maintenance of the lining of the bones and teeth	Green and yellow vegetables, yellow fruits, vegetable oils; milk and its derivatives are sources of B-carotene, which is the precursor of vitamin A (e.g. green peppers and carrots)
B	Essential in the metabolism of the cells and tissues of the muscles; also essential in protein metabolism; plays a very important role in the functioning of the nervous system	Brewer's yeast, cereals, bananas, milk, soybean oil
C	Maintains bones, teeth and blood vessels in good condition; protects against haemorraghing, colds, heart disease, cancer	Citrus fruit, kiwi, strawberries, melons, potatoes, tomatoes; green leafy vegetables, such as spinach, peppers, broccoli, etc.
D	Regulates calcium absorption from the intestine and bone tissue; essential for bone formation and development; necessary for the prevention of osteoporosis and premature ageing	Milk, mushrooms, exposure to the sun
E	Antioxidant qualities; fights inflammation and enhances the immune system	Lettuce, spinach, wholewheat bread, wheat germ

Minerals

Minerals	What they are good for	Where they are found
Calcium	Main substance in the formation of bones and teeth	Dairy products, almonds, brewer's yeast, pulses
Phosphorus	Essential for the formation of bones and teeth, cell growth and metabolism	Dairy products, asparagus, bran, carrots, cereal, corn, eggs, pulses, walnuts
Magnesium	Enzyme activity, energy production, muscles including the heart and nervous system	Dairy products, almonds, wheat germ
Potassium	Important for the functioning of muscles and nerves, maintains body's water balance	Bananas, milk, molasses, mushrooms, parsley, potatoes, pumpkin, tomatoes, white cabbage
Sodium	Maintains body's water balance, important for the muscles, nerves and stomach	Celery, miso, olives
Iron	Assists transportation of oxygen and carbon dioxide to cells, energy production	Cereals, chard, eggs, pulses (e.g. lentils), pumpkin seeds, leafy vegetables

Our health is our most valuable possession. Mother Nature's produce is the most important medicine for prevention and treatment of ill-health; it is essential for our good health, wellbeing and for strengthening the human organism.

"Purity of food leads to purity of mind."

SWAMI SIVAMURTI

"The greatest worship is Annapoorna, offering food to our fellow man."

SWAMI SATYASANGANANDA

"There are people in the world so hungry that God cannot appear to them except in the form of bread."

MAHATMA GANDHI

FIFTEEN BASIC FOODS
AND THEIR BENEFITS

Apples	rich in antioxidants
Artichokes	strengthen the liver
Carrots	sharpen vision
Cucumber	for general detoxification of the body
Garlic	regulates blood pressure; helps in existing atherosclerosis
Grapes	purify the blood
Honey	the best sedative
Onions	prevent blood clotting; strengthen the immune system
Peppers	protect against free radicals (considered responsible for many malignant diseases); red hot chilli peppers regulate and assist blood circulation
Potatoes	good for the heart and circulatory system
Radishes	increase the production of bile; help prevent gallstone formation; strengthen the liver
Spinach	important for the blood as it contains iron for the red blood cells

Tomatoes	strengthen the immune system
White cabbage	rich in vitamin B; eliminate all the ills of atherosclerosis, diabetes, intestinal diseases, heart failure
Whole grains	helps against atherosclerosis, rheumatism, arthritis and intestinal disorders

SEASONAL FRUIT AND VEGETABLES

Fruit and vegetables vary from place to place, as they are influenced by climatic conditions. Examples of fruits and vegetables found in each season are presented in the following table:

Spring	Lettuce, chard, spinach, artichokes, beetroot Strawberries, cherries
Summer	Peppers, aubergines, corn, courgettes, cucumber, green beans, okra, peas Tomatoes, peaches, apricots, mulberries, plums, kiwi, watermelon, sweet melon, grapes, figs, bananas
Autumn	Potato, red pumpkin, and everything that ripens late in the summer
Winter	Broccoli, cauliflower, carrots, cabbage, radishes, kale, leeks, onions, Brussels sprouts Pears, apples, oranges, mandarins, grapefruit

SWAMI SIVANANDA'S
DIETARY RULES

- Follow a moderate diet; in other words, the stomach should be only three-quarters full.

- Eat only when hungry.

- Do not eat between meals.

- Eat at regular hours.

- Do not eat food that is very hot or very cold.

- Include raw fruit and vegetables in your daily diet.

- Eat appropriate combinations of food.

- Avoid processed foods.

- Most fruit and vegetables do not need to be peeled.

- Do not overcook food.

- Never reheat food.

- Eat under calm conditions.

- Rest half an hour after eating.

- Avoid eating late at night.

"Food plays an important role in meditation."

SWAMI SIVANANDA

GUIDELINES FROM SWAMI SATYANANDA

- Buy fresh food and store it at a cool temperature.

- Buy food that is in season.

- Wash fruit and vegetables to remove dust and chemicals.

- Steam cooking and oven baking are preferable to boiling and frying.

- Avoid fat, oil and butter in large quantities.

- Use salt sparingly. Use herbs and spices, lemon juice and natural soy sauce.

- Avoid over-cooking and serve as soon as you have finished cooking.

- Cook with care in order to increase prana (vital energy).

- Keep meals simple.

- Eat at regular intervals without snacking in between meals.

- Chew food carefully.

- Eat when you are calm.

- Eat only as much as you need.

- Take your food with the inner attitude that it is a gift from nature, which gives us health.

"The yogi should fill two parts of the stomach with food, and the third part with water, leaving the fourth part free for air to aid digestion."

HATHA YOGA PRATIPIKA 1:58

THE RECIPES

- All the recipes make a meal for approximately four people, unless otherwise specified.

- The oil used in all the recipes is sunflower or vegetable oil. We do not generally cook with olive oil, as it is preferable to consume olive oil raw to avoid destroying its nutritional value in the heating process.

- Gram flour can also be found as garbanzo flour, which is made from raw or roasted chickpeas.

- When the recipe says to add water after you have already started cooking, this always means adding warm water to avoid temperature variations in the pot.

- The vegetables that we use are preferably fresh and organic, full of prana (vital energy).

- Ghee, an ingredient in some recipes, is "melted butter."

- Paneer, an ingredient in some recipes, is "fresh cheese" and there are instructions on to how to make it in this book (see Rasgulla recipe).

"Yogic cooking is designed in a way so that it provides energy to the body and balances the mind."

SWAMI SIVAMURTI

"The five key points to good health are: (i) being active, (ii) eating less (iii) sleeping well, (iv) maintaining a calm mind, and (v) enjoying life and yourself."

SWAMI NIRANJANANANDA

Mint Raita

- 8oz (220g) natural yogurt
- 3fl oz (80ml) water
- ½ teaspoon salt
- 1 tablespoon fresh (or dried) mint leaves, chopped

Method: Place all the ingredients in a bowl and mix well. Serve chilled.

Cucumber Raita

- 8oz (220g) natural yogurt
- 3fl oz (80ml) water
- 1 teaspoon salt
- 1 teaspoon black pepper or cayenne pepper
- 1 large cucumber, peeled and sliced into thin rounds
- 1 teaspoon cumin powder or toasted crushed cumin seeds
- 2 tablespoons fresh coriander leaves

Method: Mix the yogurt, water, salt and pepper in a bowl. Add the cucumber. Sprinkle the cumin powder or crushed cumin seeds on top. Garnish with the coriander leaves and serve chilled.

Hint: The best cumin powder to use for raita is made from seeds that have been toasted. It only takes 5 minutes to prepare your own. Sprinkle the cumin seeds into a hot frying pan and toast over a medium heat until they turn a slightly darker colour. This brings out their particular flavour. Grind to a powder.

Coconut Acha

- 8oz (220g) natural yogurt
- 3fl oz (80ml) water
- ½ teaspoon salt
- 1 teaspoon cumin seeds
- 1 teaspoon mustard seeds
- ½ teaspoon coriander seeds, crushed
- a little oil
- ½ teaspoon turmeric
- 1 or more teaspoons dessicated coconut
- 1 tablespoon finely chopped dill

Method: In a bowl mix the yogurt, water and salt.

Sauté the cumin, mustard and coriander seeds in a pan with a little oil until they begin popping. Then add the turmeric and stir for 1 minute. Add to the yogurt mixture. Stir until it becomes uniform but slightly runny. Slowly add the dessicated coconut while continuing to stir, until it becomes smooth and creamy. Add the chopped dill.

This particular acha is a wonderful accompaniment to Upma (savoury halva) and Rice Pulau (see recipes).

Red Acha

- 5–6 ripe tomatoes, finely chopped
- 3 tablespoons olive oil
- 1 teaspoon mustard seeds
- 2 teaspoons cumin seeds
- 1 teaspoon fresh ginger, grated or chopped
- ¼ teaspoon turmeric
- 2 chillies (optional)
- 1–2 cloves garlic, finely chopped
- 2 spring onions, finely chopped
- ½ teaspoon salt
- 3–4 teaspoons sugar
- 2 cloves
- 1 cinnamon stick

Method: Heat the tomatoes in a saucepan until they soften to become a sauce.

Heat the olive oil and sauté the mustard and cumin seeds, ginger, turmeric and chilli (if using). Add them to the tomato sauce, along with the garlic, onions, salt, sugar, cloves and cinnamon stick.

Stir over a low heat until the sauce thickens and most of the water has evaporated.

Yogurt Mayonnaise

- 8oz (220g) natural yogurt
- 2 teaspoons tahini (sesame paste)
- 1 teaspoon Dijon mustard
- 3fl oz (80ml) water
- pinch of salt

Method: Mix all the ingredients together until they form a smooth, thick mixture.

Hint: Beat all the ingredients in a hand mixer or blender, if you have one.

This sauce accompanies all salads and steamed vegetables.

Pineapple Chutney (or other fruit)

(MAKES 8–10 SERVINGS)

- 1 fresh, ripe pineapple
- olive oil
- 1 teaspoon mustard seeds
- 1 teaspoon cumin seeds
- 1 teaspoon fresh ginger, grated
- ½ teaspoon turmeric

- 2–3 chopped chillies (optional)
- ½ teaspoon salt
- 1 cinnamon stick
- 3–4 cloves
- 4 tablespoons brown sugar
- 1 tablespoon basil leaves, chopped

Method: Peel the pineapple and cut into small pieces.

Sauté the mustard and cumin seeds, ginger, turmeric and chillies (if using) in a frying pan with a little oil until the seeds begin popping. Add the pineapple, salt, cinnamon stick, cloves, sugar and a little water (if needed).

Boil for 20 minutes over a low heat. Before you take it off the heat, add the finely chopped basil.

Variation: This chutney can be made with ripe tomatoes or other fruit, such as apricots or mangos.

Chutney accompanies all yogic food.

Mung Beans

- 2 cups mung beans
- 2 spring onions, finely chopped
- 1 carrot, grated or finely chopped
- 1 small cup peanuts, almonds, walnuts or sunflower seeds

- juice of 1 lemon
- 2 tablespoons olive oil
- salt and pepper

Method: Soak the mung beans for 2–3 days, changing the water every day, until they sprout.

Wash them carefully until you remove most of the green skin, and put the cleaned beans in a bowl. Add all the other ingredients and mix well.

This salad is a very energizing breakfast or an accompaniment to lunch.

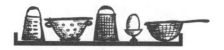

Basic Recipe

This is the basis of almost all yogic food, or accompanies it. We begin all main dishes by making the Basic Recipe, even if we keep it separately and add it at the end.

- 2–3 tablespoons oil (or ghee)
- 1 teaspoon black or white mustard seeds
- 1 teaspoon cumin seeds
- 2 medium onions, chopped
- 2–3 cloves garlic, chopped
- ½ teaspoon turmeric
- 1 teaspoon cumin powder
- 1 hot chilli pepper, or ½ teaspoon chilli powder (optional)

Method: Heat the oil in a saucepan, add the mustard and cumin seeds and stir. Once the seeds begin popping, add the onion and garlic, stirring every so often until golden brown.

Add the turmeric, cumin power and chilli (if using), stirring continuously for a few seconds.

This is your Basic Recipe.

Natural Vegetable Stock

- 1 carrot, sliced
- 1 onion, sliced
- a little celery, sliced
- 1–2 cloves (optional)
- 2½ pints (1½ litres) cold water

Method: Place the vegetables and cloves (if using) in the water and bring to the boil.

After the mixture has been boiling for 15–20 minutes, strain it and keep the clear broth. This can be used as a base for soups, gravy and more.

Béchamel Sauce

- 4 tablespoons oil
- 4 tablespoons plain flour
- 1½ pints (750ml) milk
- ½ teaspoon grated nutmeg
- salt and pepper

Method: Heat the oil and add the flour, stirring with a whisk until all the lumps dissolve. Continue stirring over a medium heat until it no longer smells "floury." Stir for another 5 minutes until the mixture begins to turn white.

Take the saucepan off the heat. Gradually add the milk, stirring continuously. If the sauce is too stiff, add a little more milk.

At the end, add the nutmeg, salt and pepper to taste.

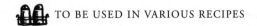

Rice

Rice is one of the staple foods of yogic cooking, which is consumed instead of wheat. Basmati rice is preferred.

Method: Pre-wash the rice thoroughly 2–3 times to rinse the starch off. Boil water and add some salt and a few drops of lemon juice, which helps the rice to stay grainy. To avoid the rice sticking, first boil the water and then add the rice. When it is ready, remove from the heat and drain.

If you like, you can add butter and chopped dill.

Dhal

Dhal is one of the most popular dishes and a rich source of protein. As a rule it is made with one type of pulse, usually with split peas, and the Basic Recipe. Dhal can also be made with mung beans, green peas or red or brown lentils.

- 1 cup split peas
- 1–2 medium onions, chopped
- 2 cloves garlic, chopped
- 2 bay leaves
- 1 quantity Basic Recipe

- salt
- 1 hot chilli pepper, chopped (optional)
- 2 tablespoons parsley, dill or coriander, finely chopped

Method: Soak the split peas overnight. The next day rinse them thoroughly in hot water. Put the split peas, onion, garlic and bay leaves in a saucepan and boil until soft and mushy and the mixture becomes smooth.

While the split pea mixture is boiling, add as much warm water as needed to prevent sticking. When the split peas are cooked, add enough warm water to make it into a thicker or thinner soup, as desired.

Put the Basic Recipe into the saucepan with the split peas and add salt. Boil once more and then remove from the heat. Add the chilli (if using), parsley, dill or coriander. The dhal is ready.

In summer, you can add a finely chopped tomato to the dhal soup.

Sambar Dhal

- 2–3 seasonal vegetables (e.g. carrot, courgette)
- oil
- 1 quantity Dhal

Method: Cut the vegetables into 1 inch cubes, and sauté in a little oil until they turn golden. Add to the dhal.

Can be served with dessicated coconut sprinkled on top.

Curry Soup

- 1lb 3oz (600g) natural yogurt
- 1 clove garlic, finely sliced
- 1 teaspoon cumin seeds
- 1 teaspoon mustard seeds
- 1 teaspoon turmeric
- 2 teaspoons salt
- 5 tablespoons gram flour
- 2½ pints (1½ litres) warm water

Method: Put the yogurt in a saucepan and stir over a low heat for a few minutes. Add the garlic, cumin and mustard seeds, turmeric and salt, stirring continuously. Slowly add the gram flour and mix until any lumps of flour dissolve. This whole process takes about 5–7 minutes. While stirring, add the water. If the mixture is too thick, add more water until it becomes more liquid. Let it simmer gently for 15 minutes over a low heat. Serve warm.

Ideal in hot weather.

Courgette Soup with Basil

- 3 onions, grated
- 2 cloves garlic, crushed
- 2 tablespoons basil leaves, finely chopped
- 3fl oz (80ml) olive oil
- 4 medium courgettes, grated
- 3 tablespoons rice (basmati or glutinous)
- ½ cup grated hard cheese (such as Greek Kefalotiri or Italian Parmesan)
- 4 cups Natural Vegetable Stock
- salt and pepper

Method: Put a little oil in a saucepan and sauté the onions, garlic and basil over a medium heat until the onions are soft. Add the courgettes, vegetable stock, salt and pepper. Stir and leave to cook for about 20 minutes.

Add the rice and leave on the heat for a further 10 minutes.

Sprinkle the cheese on top and serve.

Pumpkin Soup

- 2lb 2oz (1kg) (peeled) yellow pumpkin, seeded and chopped
- salt
- 3 tablespoons oil
- 3 cloves garlic, chopped
- 1 tablespoon fresh ginger, grated
- 1 teaspoon cumin powder
- 1 teaspoon black mustard seeds
- 3 spring onions, chopped
- 3 bull's horn peppers, chopped
- fresh parsley or dill, chopped
- chilli (optional)

Method: Put the pumpkin in water (or vegetable stock) with a little salt, and boil until it becomes soft. Add more water or stock to thin out if necessary.

In another pan add the oil and sauté the garlic and ginger until brown. Then add the cumin powder and mustard seeds for 1 minute. Pour into the soup and stir well. Add the finely chopped spring onions, bull's horn peppers, parsley or dill and chilli (if using).

Variation: If you want a richer flavour to the soup, you can add 8oz (220g) natural yogurt or 5oz (150g) double cream.

You can make potato, broccoli, carrot or leek soup in the same way.

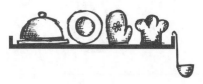

Vegetarian Magiritsa Soup

- 1 cup soya chunks
- ingredients for a simple marinade: warm water, olive oil, garlic, dried oregano
- ingredients for vegetable stock: 1 leek, sliced, 1 carrot, sliced, 1 onion, sliced and 2½ pints (1½ litres) water
- 2 large potatoes, peeled and chopped
- 3-4 tablespoons ghee or white butter

- 4–5 spring onions, finely chopped
- 1 leek, finely chopped
- salt and pepper
- 12 mushrooms, chopped
- ½ lettuce, chopped
- 1 tablespoon glutinous rice
- ¼ teaspoon ginger powder
- 1 tablespoon dill, chopped
- 5oz (150g) cream

Method: Marinate the soya overnight in a simple marinade.

Prepare a natural vegetable stock by boiling all the ingredients for 15–20 minutes until the flavour and nutrients of the vegetables are in the water. Drain the vegetables; the stock that is left will be used for the soup.

Boil the potatoes in a little water until soft. Make a smooth potato puree with a little water that has been left in the pot.

Take the soya out of the marinade, squeeze out the liquid and finely chop. Put aside the rest of the marinade as you will need it later on. Add enough ghee or butter to a pan to sauté the finely chopped soya until it turns brown. In another pan sauté the spring onions and leek in a little oil and then season. When the onions and leeks are soft, add the mushrooms and lastly add the lettuce. Stir in the soya and mix well. Add the vegetable stock, potato puree and the leftover marinade.

Add the rice and the ginger and cook for a few more minutes.

Finally, before you turn off the heat, stir in the dill and the cream and mix well.

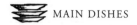

Sabji

Sabji is one of the basic dishes of yogic cooking. It usually consists of potatoes and one other vegetable, plus the Basic Recipe. The preferred vegetables for sabji are cauliflower, broccoli or courgettes.

- 4 medium potatoes, cubed
- 2–3 courgettes, sliced or one small cauliflower or broccoli, florets
- 4 tablespoons oil or ghee
- parsley or coriander
- salt
- 1 quantity Basic Recipe

Method: While preparing the Basic Recipe, put the chopped potatoes in water to keep them fresh. Do the same with the vegetables.

When the Basic Recipe is ready, add the potatoes and sauté for about 15 minutes. Add the vegetables, stir so that the Basic Recipe is totally mixed in, and continue sautéing for another 10 minutes until the vegetables are soft.

Add hot water and salt, cover the saucepan and allow the food to cook over a low heat for about 30 minutes, without stirring. Just give the saucepan a shake every now and again to prevent the food from sticking. Just before the sabji is done, you can add parsley or coriander and cover it again. To see if is ready, lightly prick a potato with a knife. If it is soft and comes apart, the sabji is ready.

Sabji is correctly prepared when the broth is clear and the vegetables are neither overdone nor mushy.

Variation: Straying a bit from the standard sabji recipe, another option is to add 1 or 2 carrots or 1 sliced green pepper.

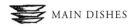

Paneer Palak

- 4–6 tablespoons olive oil
- 2 medium onions or leeks, chopped or sliced
- 2 cloves garlic, chopped
- 1 teaspoon cumin seeds
- 1 teaspoon cumin powder
- 1 teaspoon mustard seeds
- 1 teaspoon turmeric

- 2lb 2oz (1kg) spinach, washed and chopped
- 4 tablespoons parsley or coriander, finely chopped
- 8oz (220g) natural yogurt
- 7oz (200g) paneer, fried (see Rasgulla recipe for how to make your own paneer)
- salt and pepper

Method: Put the oil in a pan and lightly sauté the onions or leeks. Add the garlic and spices, season, and cook until the seeds pop. Add the spinach and parsley (or coriander) and a little water, stirring well. Leave to boil for about 15 minutes, then remove from the heat.

In a bowl, add the yogurt and beat until it becomes smooth. Then, using a wooden spoon, slowly add the liquid from the sautéed vegetables, stirring continuously to prevent curdling. When the spinach and the yogurt mixture are about the same temperature, pour the yogurt mixture back into the pot with the spinach, stirring to mix it in well.

Serve on a platter with pieces of fried paneer on top.

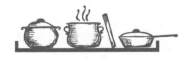

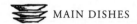

Bhaji

- 4–6 tablespoons olive oil
- 2 medium onions or leeks, chopped or sliced
- 2 cloves garlic, chopped
- 1 teaspoon cumin seeds
- 1 teaspoon cumin powder
- 1 teaspoon mustard seeds
- 1 teaspoon turmeric
- 2lb 2oz (1kg) spinach, washed and chopped
- 4 tablespoons parsley or coriander, finely chopped
- salt and pepper

Method: Make the bhaji in exactly the same way as Paneer Palak, but without the yogurt or paneer.

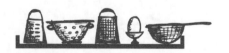

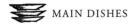

Briam (vegetable casserole)

- 4 potatoes, diced
- 1lb (½kg) aubergines, diced
- 2lb 2oz (1kg) courgettes, diced
- 2 green peppers
- 2 medium onions or 8–10 spring onions, finely chopped
- 4–5 tomatoes, chopped or grated
- 1 teaspoon sugar
- oil
- 1–2 cups water or vegetable stock
- 1 handful parsley, finely chopped
- salt and pepper

Method: Cut the potatoes, courgettes and aubergines into equal-sized pieces so that they take the same amount of time to cook. Leave the cut aubergines in salt water for about half an hour to remove the bitterness, then rinse and drain them well. Remove the seeds from the green peppers and cut into four pieces.

Place these ingredients in an oven-proof baking dish or in a casserole pot along with the onions. Add the salt, pepper, tomatoes and a pinch of sugar. Add the oil and one cup of warm water or vegetable stock. Bake in the oven at 180°C (350°F/GM4) for one hour.

If using a casserole pot, cook the food over a medium heat for about 40 minutes, depending on the size of the vegetables. Check at regular intervals that the food has enough liquid and add water as required. Stir in the parsley before serving.

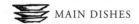

Courgette and Potato Moussaka

- 2lb 2oz (1kg) potatoes, sliced
- 2lb 2oz (1kg) courgettes, sliced
- 2–3 medium onions, chopped
- 1 cup fresh tomatoes, 400g (14oz) tinned tomatoes or 1 tablespoon tomato puree
- parsley and mint, finely chopped
- 1 handful breadcrumbs
- oil
- salt and pepper

Method: Lightly fry the potatoes and courgettes (avoid them turning brown). Place on absorbent kitchen paper to remove any excess oil. Sauté the onions in oil.

Add the tomatoes, salt, pepper and mint. Cook for 15 minutes and add a little of the breadcrumbs.

In an oven-proof baking dish layer the potatoes, followed by a layer of the tomato mixture, then a layer of courgettes, and then another layer of the tomato mixture. Continue alternating the layers, ending with the tomato mixture, a little extra oil drizzled over and some chopped parsley. Sprinkle over the rest of the breadcrumbs and place in the oven at a moderate temperature (170–180°C/340°F/GM4) until it goes golden brown on top.

Variation: Instead of breadcrumbs you can use a grated yellow cheese or crumbled feta.

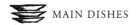

Rice Pulau

- 2 cups basmati rice
- 2 courgettes, cubed
- 1 green pepper, chopped
- 1 red pepper, chopped
- 1 yellow pepper, chopped
- 2 carrots, diced

- 1 quantity Basic Recipe
- 2–3 spring onions, finely chopped
- 2 tablespoons dill, finely chopped
- 1 cup coarsely chopped nuts (almonds, pistachios, hazelnuts or cashews)
- salt and pepper

Method: In a saucepan cook the rice (see Rice recipe) and then drain.

Sauté the courgettes, peppers and carrots. When done, place on absorbent kitchen paper. Prepare the Basic Recipe using the finely chopped spring onions to replace the onions and garlic. Mix it with the rice and the fried vegetables. Season and add the dill and nuts.

Rice Pulau is a tasty dish that can accompany every meal. This recipe makes four large servings or 8–10 smaller servings as a side dish. It is accompanied by red acha or acha with dessicated coconut.

Rice Pulau can be made with whatever vegetables you like, such as cauliflower, broccoli, green beans or aubergines.

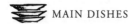

Biryani

- 2 cups vegetable stock
- 5oz (150g) basmati rice
- 5oz (150g) butter
- 2 onions, thinly sliced
- 2 teaspoons coriander powder

- 2 teaspoons cumin powder
- salt
- 1 cauliflower, florets only
- 10½oz (300g) natural yogurt
- 1 handful fresh coriander, finely chopped

Method: Prepare the vegetable stock. Wash the rice. In a saucepan melt the butter and sauté the sliced onions until transparent. Add the spices and a pinch of salt (optional), and stir for another 2 minutes. Add the cauliflower and stir for 1 minute. Add the rice and the vegetable stock. When it starts to boil, cover the pan and leave it to simmer for around 10–15 minutes, until the liquid has completely evaporated. If it has evaporated before the rice has cooked, you will need to add a little extra water.

Mix the yogurt with the fresh coriander and spoon it over the rice before serving.

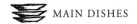

Vegetable Curry

- 2 medium courgettes, diced
- 3 bull's horn peppers or sweet long red peppers, diced
- 2 medium carrots, diced
- 3–4 tablespoons sunflower or sesame oil
- 2 medium onions, finely chopped
- 2 cloves garlic, crushed
- 1 inch (2½cm) fresh ginger, chopped or 1 teaspoon ginger powder

- 1 cinnamon stick
- 3 cardamom pods, opened
- 1 teaspoon cumin powder
- 1 teaspoon coriander powder
- 1 teaspoon curry powder
- salt
- 4 tablespoons natural yogurt
- 2 tablespoons tomato puree
- 1 cup warm water
- 2 tablespoons parsley, chopped

Method: Sauté the courgettes, peppers and carrots in a pan with oil until golden. Then drain on absorbent kitchen paper.

Heat the oil in a big pan. Add the onion, garlic, ginger, cinnamon stick and cardamom pods and cook for 5 minutes until the onion becomes soft and golden and you can smell the spices. Add the sautéed vegetables, the cumin, coriander, curry powder, a little salt, and stir thoroughly.

In another bowl mix the yogurt with the tomato puree and water. Pour into the pan and stir well. Cook for 15 minutes on a low heat, until the liquid evaporates and the sauce thickens. Before turning off the heat, add the chopped parsley.

Serve with basmati rice or a selection of breads.

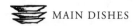

Cauliflower Au Gratin

- 1 medium cauliflower or broccoli, florets
- 2–3 medium onions, chopped
- 1 cup white cheese, grated
- 1 cup yellow cheese, grated
- 1 quantity Béchamel Sauce
- salt and pepper

Method: Boil the cauliflower or broccoli florets in salted water (if you want you can throw out the water when it first starts to boil and add fresh boiled water). Sauté the onion in a little oil in a frying pan.

Mix the cauliflower or broccoli with the sautéd onion and cheese (keep a bit of the yellow cheese to put on the Béchamel Sauce). Cover the bottom of an oven-proof baking dish with some of the béchamel sauce and sprinkle with the rest of the cheese. Put a layer of the cauliflower or broccoli in the baking dish and pour the rest of the béchamel sauce over the cauliflower, making sure it is covered.

Bake at 180°C (350°F/GM4) for 30 minutes, until it goes golden on top.

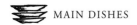

Dum Aloo (baby potatoes)

(MAKES 6 SERVINGS)

- 1 teaspoon cumin seeds
- 1 teaspoon cumin powder
- 1 teaspoon mustard seeds
- 1 teaspoon ground coriander
- ½ teaspoon turmeric
- 2 cloves garlic, crushed
- 1–2 chillies (optional)

- salt
- 4lb 4oz (2kg) medium potatoes, peeled and cut lengthwise
- 4 tablespoons olive oil
- 3fl oz (80ml) water
- 8oz (220g) natural yogurt
- 2 tablespoons parsley, mint or fresh coriander

Method: In a bowl, mix the cumin seeds, cumin powder, mustard seeds, ground coriander, turmeric, garlic, chilli and salt. Mix this into the potatoes so that they are thoroughly covered. Place the potatoes in an oven-proof baking dish, add the olive oil and the water.

Depending on the size of the potatoes, bake at 160°C (325°F/ GM3) for about 40–60 minutes, until they are golden brown. Add a little more water to prevent sticking if required.

When the potatoes are ready, turn off the oven. Beat the yogurt with a little water and pour it over the potatoes. Leave in the hot oven for another 5 minutes.

Serve sprinkled with parsley, mint or coriander.

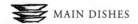

Khichari

- basmati rice
- 1 quantity Dhal
- butter or ghee

Method: Cook the basmati rice and drain.

In a pan, add 2 parts (e.g. cups) dhal to 3 parts cooked rice. Mix and add a little hot water as needed. The final mixture should be a thick soup.

Add ghee (melted butter) on top, if desired.

Khichari is a complete food source, good for the digestive system.

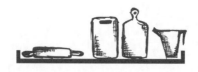

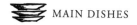

Chickpeas with Rice

(MAKES 6 SERVINGS)

- 1lb (500g) dried chickpeas
- 3 spring onions, finely chopped
- ¾ cup olive oil
- ½ cup basmati rice

- 2 tablespoons parsley, finely chopped
- chilli pepper, chopped
- juice of 1 lemon
- salt and pepper

Method: Wash the chickpeas and leave them to soak in water overnight.

Wash the chickpeas again. Bring the water to boil in a pan and add the chickpeas and the spring onions.

Cover the pan with a lid and leave to cook for around 1½ hours, until the chickpeas soften. Towards the end, add the olive oil and season and leave to boil for a few more minutes.

Cook the basmati rice and drain.

Add to the chickpeas the rice, chilli pepper, parsley and lemon juice to taste and serve.

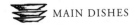

Upma

Upma is a great recipe. It can be eaten for breakfast or at any time of the day. It is also a nice snack for the road. Traditionally, the Basic Recipe for upma is made with ghee instead of oil.

- 2–3 spring onions, chopped
- 1 courgette, sliced, or broccoli or cauliflower florets
- 1 green pepper, chopped
- 1 carrot, chopped
- 3fl oz (80ml) oil
- 1½ cups coarse semolina
- salt and pepper
- pinch of sugar
- 3 cups hot water
- 1 quantity Basic Recipe
- ½ cup cashews or peanuts
- 1 handful dill, chopped (optional)

Method: Fry the spring onions and vegetables until lightly golden and then drain on absorbent kitchen paper.

Heat the oil in a pan. Cook the semolina with salt, pepper and a pinch of sugar, until it browns. Stir continuously to prevent it burning. When the semolina is golden brown, slowly pour in the hot water, stirring continuously with a wooden spatula, at a low temperature. When the semolina starts to unstick from the sides of the pan, it means that the upma is ready.

In a pan prepare the Basic Recipe and add the semolina, as well as the vegetables, the cashews or peanuts and dill (optional). Mix all the ingredients and serve.

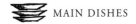

Fried Vegetable Cutlets

(MAKES 30 PIECES)

- 4–6 tablespoons oil
- 2 onions, finely chopped
- salt
- 2 cups finely chopped vegetables (carrots, cauliflower)
- ½ teaspoon coriander powder
- ½ teaspoon black pepper
- ½ teaspoon cumin powder
- ½ teaspoon cumin seeds
- ½ teaspoon nutmeg
- 1 teaspoon chat masala (optional)
- ½ teaspoon chilli powder (optional)
- 4–6 potatoes, mashed
- 1 cup gram flour (for the batter)
- 4 cups breadcrumbs

Method: Heat the oil in a saucepan and sauté the onions with a little salt. Add the vegetables, continuing to sauté. Spray with a little water if needed. Add all the spices and the chilli and chat masala, if using.

Add the mashed potatoes, continuing to sauté for a few minutes. Then place the mixture in the refrigerator to cool while you prepare the batter with the gram flour and water.

When the mixture has cooled, make cutlets in the shape of a crescent. Dip each in the batter, and then cover with breadcrumbs.

Carefully place the cutlets in the frying pan so that they don't fall apart. Fry in hot oil on one side until crusty, then turn them over. They are ready when golden brown on both sides.

Serve hot with Red Acha (see recipe).

Variation: You can also add ginger, mustard seeds or crushed garlic to the mixture.

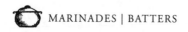

Marinades are mixtures of liquid and solid ingredients, herbs, aromatic plants, spices, and vegetables. They add flavour and fragrance to enhance the taste of each food. The quantities for the marinades are for four people or more.

Marinade for Barbecued Vegetables

- 1 cup olive oil
- ½ teaspoon dried oregano
- 1 teaspoon dried tarragon
- juice of 1 lemon
- 2–3 cloves garlic, crushed (optional)

- a selection of vegetables (e.g. aubergine, tomatoes, courgette rounds or whole mushrooms)
- salt and pepper
- packet of wooden skewers

Method: Combine all the ingredients and mix well to make a marinade. Brush the marinade onto the vegetables. Refrigerate.

After an hour, brush the marinade onto the vegetables again, and leave for another 2 hours. Skewer the vegetables onto soaked wooden skewers, and then grill or barbecue.

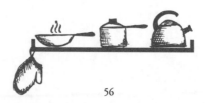

Marinade for Baked Potatoes

- 3 teaspoons wholegrain mustard
- 5 teaspoons honey, diluted in 2 tablespoons warm water
- 3 large potatoes, dried
- 3fl oz (80ml) oil
- pinch of dried oregano

Method: Mix the mustard and diluted honey to make a smooth paste. Brush onto the potatoes and chill for 2 hours. Before cooking, if necessary, brush the potatoes again with the marinade mixture or with a little oil. Bake in the oven either on a tray or in a baking dish at 170°C (340°F/GM3) for about 35 minutes.

The potatoes are ready when they are soft on the inside and golden brown on the outside. Serve hot sprinkled with oregano.

Exotic Marinade for Thai Barbecue

This marinade is for vegetables that are stir-fried in a wok (a deep round Chinese frying pan).

- 5½fl oz (160ml) soy sauce
- 1 tablespoon honey
- 1 tablespoon olive oil or sesame seed oil
- 2 tablespoons fresh ginger, grated
- 2 cloves garlic, crushed
- a selection of vegetables (e.g. carrots, leeks, courgettes, potatoes, cut into thin strips, or cauliflower or broccoli florets)

Method: In a bowl mix the soy sauce, honey, oil, ginger and garlic together, place the vegetables in the mixture and chill for 2 hours.

Heat the oil in a large pan or wok, add the vegetables and stir-fry. When they are nearly ready, add the remaining marinade.

Serve with boiled noodles or basmati rice.

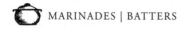

Batter for Fried Vegetables

- 2½ cups flour
- 1½ cups warm water
- 1 teaspoon baking powder
- 1 teaspoon mint, finely chopped
- 2 cloves garlic, crushed
- 1 teaspoon cumin or nutmeg powder
- seasonal vegetables of your choice
- sunflower oil

Method: Gradually add the flour to the warm water, stirring to prevent lumps. Add all the other ingredients to make a thick mixture. If you dip a piece of vegetable into the batter, it should be creamy and stiff and stick to the vegetable. Add the chopped vegetables to the batter so they sit in the mixture for at least 2 hours. Then fry them in hot sunflower oil.

Variation: Replace ½ cup water with 1 cup beer, leave out the baking powder and add a handful of dried mint or basil instead of the cumin or nutmeg, and 2 finely chopped spring onions.

Black-eyed Bean Salad

- 1lb (500g) dried black-eyed beans
- 1 medium onion or 2–3 spring onions, finely chopped
- 5fl oz (150ml) olive oil
- 2 tablespoons parsley, chopped
- juice of 1 lemon
- salt

Method: Cook the black-eyed beans in plenty of water for 5 minutes. Once they have just started to boil, drain them. Then fill the pot with cold water and start boiling them again. Be careful that the beans do not overboil and start to go mushy. Drain well and tip into a salad bowl. Mix the onion and parsley in with the beans. Add the olive oil and lemon juice, and salt to taste.

Variation: You can add one or more of the following: diced and seeded tomatoes, raw grated courgettes or pieces of blanched courgettes, finely chopped green pepper, grated carrot, fresh oregano, or grated cucumber.

Lentil Salad

- ½ cup rice
- 1 small onion, finely chopped
- 1 bay leaf
- 1 large cup lentils
- 1 tablespoon apple cider vinegar
- ½ cup olive oil
- ½ teaspoon coriander powder
- ½ teaspoon cumin powder
- salt and pepper
- 1 bunch parsley, chopped

Method: Boil the rice in a pot with a little water.

In another pot, add the onion and bay leaf and boil the lentils in enough water to cover.

To make the vinaigrette, mix the apple cider vinegar, olive oil, coriander and cumin together in a small bowl, and season to taste. Stir well and leave it to one side.

When the lentils and the rice are cooked, drain well and while still in the strainer cool under cold running water.

Mix the lentils and the rice together and put on a platter. Pour the vinaigrette dressing over and chill. Before serving, garnish with the finely chopped parsley and some pepper.

Variation: The same salad can be made with small white beans, chickpeas, or mung beans.

PULSES

Moogoris (vegetarian falafel)

- 1 cup split peas (soaked overnight)
- 5½fl oz (160ml) olive oil
- 1 quantity Basic Recipe
- 1 medium onion, chopped
- 1 teaspoon baking powder
- 3½oz (100g) wholemeal flour
- 4 tablespoons parsley, dill or mint, chopped

- ½ teaspoon turmeric
- 1 teaspoon black mustard seeds
- 1 teaspoon cumin powder
- 1 teaspoon cumin seeds
- 1 teaspoon peppercorns or red or green chilli peppers (optional)
- ½ cup breadcrumbs

Method: Put the split peas in a blender or small mixer with the oil and beat to a smooth texture.

In a pan prepare the Basic Recipe.

Mix all the ingredients together to make a tight stiff dough. Knead into a uniform dough. Add more breadcrumbs and oil as needed to get the desired texture. Shape into small balls, cover in flour and fry in hot oil.

Variation: Instead of split peas, you can use mung beans or chickpeas.

Works well accompanied by Raita, Yogurt Mayonnaise or Red Acha (see recipes).

BREADS

The bread of yogis are chapatti, roti (otherwise known as naan), puri and paratha roti.

Chapattis

(MAKES 10 PIECES)

- 1 cup white flour
- pinch of salt
- 1 teaspoon oil
- warm water, as needed
- butter or ghee for brushing

Method: In a bowl mix the flour and salt, gradually adding the oil and the water, stirring and kneading with your hands to make a smooth, soft dough. Cover the dough and leave to settle for an hour.

On a lightly floured board divide the dough into pieces the size of a walnut and roll into balls. Press each ball in your hands to flatten. With a rolling pin, sprinkle a little flour on the dough and roll out to the size of a saucer, about 2mm thick, making the circle as round as possible.

Heat a stainless steel, heavy-bottomed pan (without oil) over a low heat. When the pan is hot enough, put the chapattis in, one at a time. When bubbles begin to appear on one side, turn it over and cook the other side – about 20 seconds each side.

Hold the chapatti with a pair of tongs directly over an open flame for a few seconds until it puffs up. Then turn it over and do the same on the other side. The chapatti will be covered in brown spots. (Do not get discouraged if you don't make the chapatti puff up every time – this takes practice.)

While the chapatti is hot, and before you serve it, you can brush it with a little butter or ghee.

Keep the chapattis warm in a bread basket, covered with a clean teatowel.

Variation: Replace the flour with 2 cups wholemeal flour, and mix ⅓ cup natural yogurt into the dough.

Puri

(MAKES 10 PIECES)

- 1 cup white flour
- 1 cup wholemeal flour
- ⅓ cup ghee
- warm water, as needed
- extra ghee or oil for frying

Method: In a bowl mix the flours, ghee and water. Knead for 3 minutes. Divide the dough into pieces the size of a walnut and roll into balls. Press each ball in your hands to flatten it. With a rolling pin, sprinkle a little flour on the dough and roll out to the size of a saucer, about 2mm thick, making the circle as round as possible.

Heat the ghee or oil in a wok or a deep frying pan. The ghee has to be very hot. Cook one puri at a time. It will sink to the bottom when you first place it in the pan and then float and puff up. Cook on both sides until the puri is a golden colour. This takes about 45 seconds. (Do not be discouraged if they don't always puff up.)

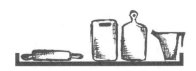

Roti

(MAKES 1 PIECE)

- 1 cup white flour
- pinch of salt
- 1 teaspoon oil
- warm water, as needed
- butter or ghee for brushing

Method: Make the dough exactly as in the Chapattis recipe but, instead of dividing the dough into balls, roll out one large roti (as big as a large frying pan), brush it with oil or ghee, and fry in a pan until golden on both sides.

Parathas Roti

(MAKES 2 PIECES)

- 1 cup white or wholemeal flour
- 1 teaspoon salt
- 1 teaspoon brown sugar
- oil or ghee
- warm water, as needed

Method: In a bowl add the flour, salt and sugar and stir. Add some oil and water, mixing and kneading with your hands to make a smooth dough. Cover and leave the dough to settle for an hour.

On a lightly floured board divide the dough into two balls and with a rolling pin, sprinkle a little flour on the dough and roll out each ball into a circle about 6 inches (15cm) in diameter. Brush the top with a little oil or ghee. Wrap it into a cylinder and make it into a ball again. Leave the dough to rest for 15 minutes and then once more, roll the dough out into a circle of about 6 inches (15cm) in diameter.

Heat some oil in a pan and cook the paratha, turning it many times.

Variation: When the dough has been rolled out the second time, you can cut it on one side and add a filling such as potato puree, and cook it like a bourek (filled pastry).

Samosas

Filling

- 2 cups cauliflower, small pieces
- 1 cup peas
- 3 tablespoons oil or ghee
- 1 green chilli, grated
- 1 teaspoon black mustard seeds
- 1 teaspoon cumin seeds
- ½ teaspoon turmeric
- 1 teaspoon garam masala
- 1 teaspoon coriander powder
- 1 teaspoon fresh ginger, grated
- ½ teaspoon salt

Pastry

- 1 cup white flour
- 1 cup wholemeal flour
- ⅓ cup of oil or ghee
- warm water, as needed (probably about ½ cup)

Method: To make the filling, boil the cauliflower and the peas until soft. Heat the oil or ghee in a pan. Add the chilli, black mustard seeds, cumin seeds, turmeric, garam masala and coriander powder.

When they start to go brown, add the ginger. Then add the boiled vegetables and 3 tablespoons of water and cook over medium heat until it becomes a thick mixture for the filling. This takes about 20 minutes. Leave it to cool.

To make the pastry, mix the flours and add ⅓ cup of oil or ghee. Add some water (about ½ a cup) and knead all the ingredients together until you get a dough with a uniform texture. The dough is ready when it no longer sticks to your hands (you may need to add a little more flour).

To assemble the samosas, divide the dough into 12 balls. Roll each ball out into a circle about 8 inches (12cm) in diameter. Cut them in half to form a crescent. In the centre of each crescent place a heaped spoonful of the filling. Fold the crescents in the middle and close by pinching the sides together, forming a triangular-shaped pyramid. Press around the edges to seal so that the samosas remain closed when frying.

Heat the oil or ghee until it is moderately hot. Add the samosas and fry until golden brown (15–20 minutes), occasionally turning and shaking to avoid any sticking. Serve hot.

Pakora

(MAKES 40–45 PIECES)

- 1 potato, grated
- 1 large onion, sliced
- 1 small cauliflower, sliced
- 3 lettuce leaves (or a small amount of cabbage or spinach or courgette, or a combination of all of these), chopped
- 1 teaspoon cumin powder
- 1 teaspoon turmeric
- ½ teaspoon chilli (optional)
- ½ handful fenugreek (optional)
- warm water
- 15oz (450g) chickpea flour
- 1 cup of sunflower oil
- salt

Method: Put all the vegetables in a bowl and add the spices. Slowly add some warm water and the chickpea flour, and knead all the ingredients together into a thick dough.

Heat the oil, take a small quantity (about the size of an apricot) of pakora in your hand, and drop it into the hot oil.

Pakora with Cauliflower

- 1 medium cauliflower, cut into pieces
- 1 cup flour
- 1 cup water
- ½ teaspoon salt
- 1 teaspoon coriander powder
- pinch of chilli powder
- ½ teaspoon turmeric
- 1 teaspoon garam masala
- oil

Method: In a bowl mix the flour and spices. Add water to make a moderately thick batter.

Heat the oil in a wok or frying pan until hot. Dip the cauliflower pieces into the batter and place in the hot oil. They will sink to the bottom of the wok and then they will rise. Fry for 5 minutes and stir until they become a dark golden colour.

Serve with Red Acha (see recipe).

Variation: This recipe can also be made with potatoes, aubergines or courgettes that have been cut into small pieces.

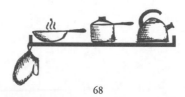

Kachori (pancakes)

- 1 cup white flour
- ½ cup gram flour
- 1 teaspoon baking powder
- 1 teaspoon cumin powder
- 1 teaspoon black mustard seeds
- ½ teaspoon turmeric
- salt
- 1 medium onion, pureed
- 2–3 cloves garlic, pureed
- warm water, as needed
- parsley or coriander

Method: Puree the onion and the garlic in a mortar or small mixer.

In a large bowl add the flours, baking powder, cumin, mustard, turmeric, salt and the pureed onion and garlic. Mix the ingredients with water until they become a soft dough. Chill for 30 minutes.

Make the dough into round balls, pat them down to flatten and fry in hot oil until golden.

Serve with chutney (see Chutney recipe) and parsley or coriander.

Variation: Add a handful of grated cheese to the dough.

Kachori with Spinach

- 1lb (500g) spinach, washed and chopped
- 1 cup white flour
- ½ cup gram flour
- 1 teaspoon baking powder
- 1 teaspoon cumin powder
- 1 teaspoon black mustard seeds
- ½ teaspoon turmeric
- 1 medium onion, pureed
- 2–3 cloves garlic, pureed
- chilli (optional)
- salt and pepper
- warm water, as needed
- oil

Method: Mix the spinach, flours, baking powder, cumin, mustard, turmeric, pureed onion, garlic and chilli (if using) and season. Stir well and pour in enough warm water to make a soft dough. Chill for 2 hours.

After you remove the mixture from the refrigerator, because the spinach releases liquid, you may want to add some more flour to stiffen the dough. To prevent the dough from sticking to your hands, rub some oil on them, make the dough into balls and roll them in flour. Fry them in hot oil until golden.

Variation: To make rice rissoles, replace the spinach with 2–3 cups of boiled rice and a cup of cheese.

To make moogori or falafel, replace the spinach with pulped split peas or chickpeas.

Sweet Halva

(FOR 6–8 PEOPLE)

- 4 cups water
- 3 cups sugar
- 1 cinnamon stick
- 1 handful whole almonds
- 1 handful raisins

- 2–3 cloves
- 1 cup oil
- 2 cups semolina
- cinnamon powder or dessicated coconut

Method: Boil the water with the sugar, cinnamon stick, almonds, raisins and cloves.

Heat the oil in a saucepan, add the semolina, cook slowly over a low heat until golden, stirring continuously to avoid burning.

When the semolina is a golden brown colour, add the warm water mixture slowly, stirring continuously.

After all the water has been soaked up, leave it to cool and serve with cinnamon powder or dessicated coconut sprinkled on top.

Rasgulla

(MAKES 12 PIECES)

Paneer (fresh cheese)

- 4 cups milk

- 2 tablespoons lemon juice with 1 tablespoon water

Syrup

- 4½ cups water

- 1½ cups sugar

Method: To make the paneer, boil the milk over a low heat and stir occasionally to avoid burning.

Once the milk starts to bubble up, gradually add the lemon juice and water mix. The mixture should begin to curdle.

Turn the heat off after 4–5 minutes and pour the mixture into a cheesecloth over a bowl. Run cold water over the mixture to wash away the taste of lemon and to facilitate the draining. Then tighten the cheesecloth and squeeze the mixture several times until all the water has been removed.

Pour the paneer onto a board, rub it and knead it for a few minutes until it thickens like soft dough. Divide it into 12 equal pieces and shape into balls with your hands.

(Variation: You can add 1 tablespoon of fine semolina in the paneer so that the dough thickens better.)

Now make the syrup. Warm the water and sugar in a medium-sized pan or a pressure cooker. Stir a little so that the sugar melts. (You can add 2 cloves and 3–4 cardamom seeds in the water with the sugar if desired.)

Before the water starts to boil, add the paneer balls. Allow to boil in a saucepan (about 30 minutes) or pressure cooker (7 minutes). The rasgulla should double in size.

Transfer the rasgulla, including the syrup, from the pan/pressure cooker into a bowl and chill them in the fridge for a few hours to ratify. Before putting them in the refrigerator, you can put a peeled and roasted almond in the heart of every rasgulla if desired.

Rice Pudding

- 1 cinnamon stick
- 7 cardamom seeds, crushed
- 3½oz (100g) sugar
- 18fl oz (500ml) milk
- 2oz (50g) glutinous rice
- 1 tablespoon corn flour

Method: In a saucepan, boil the spices in a cup of water and then add the sugar. Drain and pour the spicy liquid into the milk.

Wash the rice and boil it until al dente. Drain and keep the liquid in case you need it later.

Dissolve the corn flour in a little of the milk and then top up with water.

Boil the rest of the milk and add the prepared rice to the mixture, stirring continuously until it is cooked.

Near the end, add the corn flour mix so that the rice thickens.

Serve in individual bowls with a little cinnamon powder sprinkled on top.

Samadhi Express

- 1 tin sweetened condensed milk
- 9oz (250g) digestive biscuits
- 5oz (150g) unsalted butter
- whipped cream (optional)

Method: In a pan with water, boil the unopened tin of sweetened condensed milk for 3 hours. If the initial amount of water evaporates, don't forget to add hot water every now and then to top it up.

Leave the butter out of the refrigerator for an hour to soften.

Crush the biscuits in a bowl or tied up in a cloth until they become powder. Mix the butter and the biscuits together into a uniform base. Spread the base, about 2mm thick, on a tray that is at least 2 inches (5cm) deep. Then put the tray in the refrigerator for at least one hour.

After having boiled the tin of sweetened condensed milk, open it carefully and pour into a bowl. Stir until you have a uniform cream – it will be brown in colour as the sweetened milk will have caramelized as it boiled.

Remove the tray from the refrigerator and pour the condensed milk over the biscuit base. Again, put the tray in the refrigerator for several hours.

Before serving, you can garnish with whipped cream.

Garam Chai

It is beneficial to drink this when you have a cold.

- 1¾ pints (1 litre) water
- 1 teaspoon black tea leaves
- 2–3 mint leaves
- 2–3 leaves mountain tea
- 1 teaspoon fresh ginger, grated
- 3 cloves
- 1 cinnamon stick
- 3–4 cardamom pods
- pinch of nutmeg
- 1 chilli
- 3–4 teaspoons sugar

Method: Boil all the ingredients in a saucepan for 20 minutes. Strain and serve.

Indian Chai

This is the drink of yogis. It is served in the morning and in the afternoon. It acts as a natural digestive, it is energising, antiseptic and helps concentration.

- 1¾ pints (1 litre) water
- 2 cloves, crushed
- ½ cinnamon stick
- 1–2 cardamom pods, opened
- 3–4 level tablespoons black tea leaves
- 1–2 teaspoons sugar per person

Method: In a saucepan boil the water with the spices. When the water has boiled, turn off the heat and add the tea. Cover the saucepan and leave for precisely 3 minutes, just enough time for the mixture to get flavour and colour. Strain, add sugar as desired and serve.

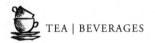

Masala Chai Tea (Indian Chai with milk)

- 1¾ pints (1 litre) milk
- 6–8 cardamom pods, opened
- 1 cinnamon stick
- 2–3 cloves
- 2–3 teaspoons black tea leaves
- 1–2 teaspoons sugar per person

Method: In a saucepan, boil the milk together with the spices. When the milk starts to bubble up, sprinkle over the black tea leaves. Leave on the heat for 1 minute and then turn off the heat. Add the sugar and stir in. Strain and serve.

Lassi

- 1lb (440g) natural yogurt
- 2½ pints (1½ litres) water
- 2 cardamom pods, opened
- 1 cinnamon stick
- 2 tablespoons sugar

Method: Dilute the yogurt in the water and stir well. Add the spices and the sugar, and stir. Leave the mixture in the refrigerator for 15 minutes.

Variation: Add 1 teaspoon of salt in place of the spices and sugar. You can also add thinly sliced fruit.